Alzheimer's Care

The Caregiver's Guide to
Understanding Alzheimer's Disease &
Best Practices to Care for People with
Alzheimer's & Dementia

Nancy J. Wiles

Alzheimer's Care

Publisher: Living Plus Healthy Publishing

ISBN-13: 978-1514251508

ISBN-10: 1514251507

Disclaimer

The Publisher has strived to be as accurate and complete as possible in the creation of this book. While all attempts have been made to verify information provided in this publication, the Publisher assumes no responsibility for errors, omissions, or contrary interpretation of the subject matter herein. Any perceived slights of specific persons, peoples, or organizations are unintentional.

This book is not intended for use as a source of legal, business, accounting or financial advice. All readers are advised to seek services of competent professionals in the legal, business, accounting, and finance fields.

The information in this book is not intended or implied to be a substitute for professional medical advice, diagnosis or treatment. All content contained in this book is for general information purposes only. Always consult your healthcare provider before carrying on any health program.

Table of Contents

Introduction

Alzheimer's disease is a common, irreversible brain disease that progressively destroys one's ability to remember and think clearly so that simple tasks become difficult or impossible to do. The usual onset of Alzheimer's dementia is about age 60. It is the most common dementia among the aged.

Dementia of any kind involves the loss of cognitive abilities so that thinking, reasoning, personality and remembering become impaired. It interferes with daily activities and the ability to take care for oneself. Dementia can be extremely mild and interfere with memory only or can be so severe that the individual needs help with even the most basic of needs like eating and toileting.

In 1906, Dr. Alois Alzheimer had a female patient who had memory problems, language difficulties and problems with behavior. He examined her brain after her death and noted what we now call amyloid plaques, which were abnormal clumps of tissue, and neurofibrillary tangles, which were tangled bundles of fibers. These are the major brain features of Alzheimer's dementia. In addition to these features, the brain loses its connections between the various nerve fibers.

No one knows exactly what triggers Alzheimer's disease to begin. We do know that evidence for the disease in the elderly can be seen up to ten years before symptoms begin. Changes are taking place in the brain even as the person continues to function normally. When the neurons become affected, the brain doesn't function as well as it used to.

When the hippocampus becomes affected by Alzheimer's disease, the person becomes unable to form new memories and recent memory becomes seriously impaired. The brain then begins to shrink and, over time, the damage becomes widespread throughout the brain.

Statistics on Alzheimer's Disease

More than 5 million US citizens have Alzheimer's disease today and, in the absence of a cure or prevention, the number will likely increase to between 11 million and 16 million by the year 2050. It affects about 13 percent of individuals over the age of 65 and about 50 percent of those over the age of 85. Almost 15 million Americans spend their time caring for a person with Alzheimer's dementia.

Between the years 2000 and 2006, the deaths related to stroke, prostate cancer and heart decreased by about 12-18 percent; however, the death rate of Alzheimer's disease patients has increased by about 66 percent.

The Science of Alzheimer's Disease

Researchers have been doing studies on the brains of people with Alzheimer's disease in an attempt to understand plaques, neurofibrillary tangles and other things found in the disease. They can now identify these brain structures in living people, especially the beta-amyloid deposits. They are trying to understand the basis behind getting these brain changes. They want to know what exactly causes the disease.

Researchers are trying to figure out why mostly older adults are affected by Alzheimer's disease. They are looking at the normal changes that occur in the aging brain and how this differs from abnormal changes. They believe that normal age-related alterations in the brain can actually do harm to the brain so that Alzheimer's can develop. Normal age-related changes include shrinking of the brain, brain inflammation, and the formation of free radicals, unstable molecules that do damage to cells. The mitochondria may also be affected and be unable to make the proper amount of energy for brain cells.

Researchers are also studying early-onset Alzheimer's disease, which is rare but believed to be hereditary. People get this form of the disease between 30 and 60 years of age; they represent only about 5 percent of all cases of Alzheimer's disease. It is a familial form of the disease, inherited from at least one parent.

Most people, on the other hand, have late onset Alzheimer's dementia and it starts at around 60 years of age. Many researchers have connected the APOE gene or "apolipoprotein" gene that comes in 4 forms. Apolipoprotein E4 appears to be connected to getting Alzheimer's disease. Interestingly, if you have this form of the gene, you don't necessarily get the disease. Experts believe you need more than one gene to cause late onset Alzheimer's disease and that APOE E4 is just one of them.

Other researchers are looking into lifestyle factors and how they play a role in getting Alzheimer's dementia. It seems to be related to the same things that give you stroke, high blood pressure, heart disease, obesity and diabetes. They are trying to understand the interrelationships between these diseases and dementia. A nutritious diet seems to help as well as good social environments, excellence in mental pursuits and plenty of physical activity. Researchers are studying these factors as they relate to Alzheimer's dementia as we speak.

Summary

Alzheimer's dementia is relatively common as brain diseases go and, as the nation's population ages, there will be more people with the disease, even double or more. Alzheimer's dementia affects thinking, memory, and behavior so that the severe Alzheimer's patient needs help with most, if not all, activities of daily living. It is up to the caregiver to do these things for the affected patient and to

help them do as much as they can by themselves or with assistance.

In the next chapter, we'll talk more about
the causes of Alzheimer's disease so you can
see the science behind the person who suffers
from the disease.

Chapter 1: Causes of Alzheimer's Disease

In truth, no one knows the exact cause of Alzheimer's disease but they do know it results from a mixture of lifestyle habits, genetic factors and environmental concerns that, over time, affect the brain.

It is caused solely by genetic factors less than five percent of the time. More likely, the disease is caused by changes in the genetic profile that predisposes someone to develop the disease. Early onset Alzheimer's disease is the only aspect of the disease that is more than likely to be completely hereditary.

Regardless of the cause, researchers do know that Alzheimer's disease does damage to and kills brain cells. Autopsies show that patients with Alzheimer's disease have fewer brain cells and fewer connections between brain cells than people without the disease. As the brain cells die, the patients have a significantly smaller brain due to shrinkage.

There are two findings that doctors and researchers see in the Alzheimer's brain that are not seen in normal brains. They seem to be hallmarks of the disease but exactly how they get there is not clear.

- **Plaques**. These are clumps of abnormal protein known as beta-amyloid. The plaques interfere with the communication between cells, which may be why the cell to cell communication is so poor.

- **Tangles**. Also called neurofibrillary tangles, these threads of tau protein become twisted into tangled shapes, interfering with the transport system of nutrients inside the brain and interfering with the brain's support system. The tangles show up inside the cells of the brain so the transport system fails. It is believed to be one way that cells die in Alzheimer's disease.

Risk Factors

Even though we don't know the exact causes of Alzheimer's disease, certain risk factors are known. Just because you have these risk factors, however, doesn't mean that you'll definitely get the disease. The risk factors include:

- **Age**. While Alzheimer's disease generally begins around age 60, the risk of getting the disease doubles every five years after the age of 65. Certain young people, as young as 30, can get the disease in a heritable way. The risks are as follows: Between the ages of 65 and 75, 1 in 100 gets the disease. Between the ages of 75 and 84, one in 14 exhibits the disease. Above age 85, the risk of getting the disease is up to one in four.

- **Family history**. It turns out that if you have a close relative who had Alzheimer's disease, you have a slightly greater risk of getting the disease, too. The risk is higher but not too high. Only seven percent of Alzheimer's patients have a truly heritable disease and this is the early-onset disease we've talked about.

- **Down syndrome**. If you have Down syndrome, you carry an extra copy of a gene related to Alzheimer's disease on chromosome 21. This puts you at a greater risk of getting the disease because you have more of the protein that causes it.

- **Aluminum**. There is a theory that excesses of aluminum are related to getting Alzheimer's disease. This is because aluminum exists in the plaques and tangles within the brain. Unfortunately, there has been no clear research indicating that aluminum excess triggers Alzheimer's disease.

- **Whiplash or head injuries**. Having either of these two events happening to you can increase your risk of developing Alzheimer's disease.

- **Gender**. From research, it has been discovered that women get Alzheimer's disease more commonly that men. Part of this is because women tend to live longer than men.

- **Having cognitive impairment**. If you were born with or have impairment of memory as a baseline, you are likely to develop Alzheimer's disease. Some believe that having mild cognitive impairment is just a case of having early Alzheimer's disease.

- **Atrial fibrillation**. One study that looked at 37,000 patients found that having atrial fibrillation puts one at risk for developing Alzheimer's disease.

- **Heart disease**. Patients who have high blood pressure, high cholesterol, or diabetes that isn't in good control have a higher than average risk of getting Alzheimer's disease. It appears that eating a healthy diet, exercising a lot, sleeping at least 7-8 hours of sleep per night, and being of a healthy body weight are ways to circumvent this risk.

- **Academic level**. This link appears to be valid. People with low educational qualifications tend to be at risk for Alzheimer's disease when compared to individuals who are highly educated.

- **Nitrates in processed foods**. Nitrates in processed foods and in fertilizer have been linked to getting Alzheimer's disease. They can also cause an increased risk of Parkinson's disease and diabetes. The study looked into increasing exposure of humans to nitrites and nitrates, found in fertilizers and preserved foods.

- **Other conditions that increase the risk**. These include having depression, having certain chronic inflammatory disorders, a history of strokes and obesity.

Summary

While researchers do not yet know the cause or causes of Alzheimer's disease, there are specific findings on pathology that can be studied and numerous risk factors for the condition that can help doctors focus on an ultimate cause that can be controlled so that one day, Alzheimer's disease can be prevented.

Chapter 2: Stages of Alzheimer's Disease

Alzheimer's disease can look like a lot of things. It can be the lonely elderly woman with mild memory impairment who can still live in her home. It can be the elderly, ambulatory, confused man who needs to live in the care of relatives. It can also be the non-ambulatory, nonverbal woman who needs help with all her cares. This is why we say that Alzheimer's disease progresses in stages with, with some stages being hardly noticeable.

Alzheimer's disease usually develops slowly and gets worse on a gradual basis over several years. It affects primarily the memory, judgment, language, thinking, personality, movement and ability to problem-solve. People with Alzheimer's disease live, on average, about 8-10 years after being diagnosed with the disease; however, there are others that live up to 25 years post-diagnosis. Common causes of death include pneumonia, which happens due to an inability to swallow foods and fluids well. Other causes of death include falls and urinary tract infections.

There are many stages of Alzheimer's disease that are unique in the amount and degree of impairment. Understanding the stages of the disease can help you and your family members know where your loved one is at in the process. It helps you plan for the future and to know what treatments can best help your loved one at the stage things are at.

Preclinical Disease

In reality, Alzheimer's dementia begins many years before the symptoms become apparent. You wouldn't notice anything if you were going to get the disease and no one around you will notice anything. Special brain tests, however, would be able to show the presence of amyloid deposits in your brain. This stage lasts a long time—up to several decades.

The most important thing about this stage of the disease is that, when new treatments for Alzheimer's disease are developed, people can possibly be treated before they develop symptoms and no one would have to endure the pain of the disability.

Mild Cognitive Impairment

Those with mild cognitive impairment have minimal changes in thinking and memory. While they're noticeable, the changes don't affect work or family relationships at this point. The sufferer may have lapses in memory for things that are usually easily remembered. They may forget conversations, appointments or recent events. They may not be able to judge how long it takes to perform a project or may forget the project sequence. This is a person who may not be able to make sound decisions about his or her life and people will begin to notice.

Mild Dementia

During the mild stage is when most people get the diagnosis of "Alzheimer's dementia". The doctor needs to decide if the problem is really due to dementia or to a case of profound depression as this also affects memory and cognition. If due to Alzheimer's disease, the dementia only progresses.

Common symptoms of mild dementia include:

- Difficulty with problem solving, especially of complex tasks. The patient may not be able to balance a checkbook, make financial decisions or plan an event.

- There are lapses in judgment. The patient may wear inappropriate clothing for the weather and may make driving mistakes.

- There is a loss of memory, usually for recent events. New information becomes difficult to learn and the sufferer may ask the same questions over and over again, not able to retain the answer.

- Personality changes are common. People can be more withdrawn especially in social situations that challenge their memory. They may be angry out of the ordinary or have a poor attention span and poor motivation to accomplish tasks.

- Problems organizing thoughts and expressing themselves. They may have word-finding difficulties and cannot clearly express ideas they want to get across.

- Misplacing belongings or getting lost themselves. They may drive to the store only to get lost on the way, even if it was a commonly used store. Things they put down can't be found again, even if in their home.

Moderate Dementia

There is an increased need for help with activities of daily living and self-care. Common symptoms include:

- Extreme poor judgment and confusion over even simple things. They can lose track of the days of the week, the seasons and where they are. They often can't identify their own things and may take things from others that don't belong to them because they don't realize it's not theirs. Sufferers don't often know where they are unless they are in their own home.

- They can confuse family members with one another or mistake a stranger for family members. They wander around, looking for more familiar surroundings. This is what makes it so unsafe for these people to live independently.

- Memory loss becomes more profound. They lose the specific details of their current personal history such as their phone number or address. Details of their past are more preserved because they are stored in long term memory. They turn to confabulation or making up things to fill in the memory gaps.

- As for personal assistance, they might need help choosing matching clothing or clothing appropriate for the weather and occasion. They might need help with grooming, bathing, toileting and other aspects of self-care. They can have problems with losing control of bowel movements or urination.

- Personality and behavioral changes worsen. They can be really suspicious and paranoid because they don't understand what's going on around them.

They can have hallucinations—both auditory and visual hallucinations. This can drive them to become agitated or restless, especially in the late afternoon and evening.

- They can have outbursts of behavior that is both aggressive and physical.

Severe Dementia

Mental status continues its steady downhill path and things like movement and physical abilities become difficult to do on their own. Some things you'll notice:

- The sufferer can no longer communicate in a coherent fashion. Conversation becomes impossible and they can say only a few words or phrases.

- Personal cares cannot be done so that they need total assistance with things like dressing, eating, toileting and other aspects of life care.

- They may have an inability to walk on their own or even to sit up straight without pillows or other devices for assistance. They may not even be able to hold their head up. Swallowing, bladder and bowel control are lost.

The Seven Stage Diagnostic Framework

Some doctors and researchers use the seven stage diagnostic framework to define seven stages of Alzheimer's dementia. Alzheimer's patients take from 8-10 years to get through all the stages but some take up to twenty years or so.

Stage One: No Actual Impairment

In this stage, there is no memory loss and no memory impairment. The diagnosis can only be made using specialized imaging tests of the brain.

Stage Two: Minimal Impairment

Memory losses are slight and may seem to be a normal aspect of the aging process. These kinds of cognitive or memory slips happen to fifty percent of people over the age of 65 years. There may be some word-finding difficulties and memory lapses such as where the person left their keys, where they left their glasses or a phone number of a friend.

Stage Three: Early Confusional State—lasts 2-7 years

This stage is when Alzheimer's disease is finally diagnosable. Normal activities of daily living go okay but in foreign circumstances, they get confused or embarrassed. Planning, organizing, and short term memory become more obviously impaired to friends and family. Can't always understand the meaning of written paragraphs and can't learn new tasks. Things become more chaotic and disorganized in their life. They patient may be depressed or anxious because of these cognitive changes.

Stage Four: Moderate Cognitive Decline—lasts about 2 years

The diagnosis is easy to make at this point. The patient is aware of herself or himself and can identify familiar faces. Has a limited memory of present personal history and cannot manage bills or do number exercises in their head. Things like counting backward by threes from a hundred become impossible to do. The understanding of recent events is limited and the person becomes more withdrawn from social conversations or anything that will show off their limitations. The person can be really defensive about their difficulty and may need help with complex aspects of daily living.

Stage Five: Moderately Severe Cognitive Decline—lasts about 18 months

The patient has further cognitive decline and cannot live independently anymore due to the need for assistance in activities of daily living. Don't remember as many details of past or present personal history and are confused as the day of the week, the month or the seasons. There is a serious impairment of mathematical skills and they need assistance with selecting the right clothing for the season and getting it on correctly. Daily living tasks may need to be assisted but usually can toilet themselves and know the names of close family members.

Stage Six: Severe Cognitive Decline — lasts about 2 1/2 years

Memory worsens and personality changes greatly. Care for personal cares needed round the clock. The patient is unaware of all present experiences and has no short term memory. Can't recall personal statistics but can usually remember their name. Can only recognize close family members but cannot name them. They are able to nonverbally express pain and pleasure but cannot dress themselves. They may be unable wash themselves and are incontinent of bowel and bladder. They usually need help with the hygiene aspects of toileting. Sleep patterns are no longer normal and they often wander off, not knowing where they are. They become very paranoid of others, especially of caregivers. They repeat normal words or nonsense syllables and engage in repetitive or compulsive types of behavior like wringing hands. They can be disturbed or agitated, especially late in the day. Hallucinations involving sight, hearing and smell are common, especially late in the day. They can often still respond to nonverbal stimuli.

Stage Seven: Very Severe Cognitive Impairment—lasts 1 to 2 1/2 year

This is a person who cannot respond to the environment but is nonverbal and does not respond to commands. Movement cannot be controlled and all care is because of a caregiver's aid. They have severe limitations of their cognitive ability and cannot speak or recognize speech. They eventually lose the ability to walk, then sit and then hold their head up. They lose the ability to smile. They undergo a failure of body systems and have swallowing difficulties. Their deep tendon reflexes are abnormal and some can suffer from seizures. The muscles stiffen as they become bedridden. They tend to sleep a lot and definitely need 24 hour care.

Summary

Regardless of the classification system you use, you can see where there is a steady progression from memory slips to behavioral changes and an inability to partake in activities of daily living. The Alzheimer's patient loses the ability to speak and recognize speech and eventually has motor problems that lead to them being wheelchair bound or bedridden. They eventually need total care, including eating and toileting and must be cleaned and dressed by trained staff.

The total duration of the disease is about 10 years although some people can have amyloid plaques and neurofibrillary tangles and no clinical disease for many years. This is the most variable part of the disease course.

Chapter 3: Safety in the Care of Alzheimer's Patients

One of the most important factors you need to consider when taking care of an Alzheimer's patient is safety. Because of their memory impairment and lack of judgment, they often make safety mistakes that can yield injuries such as lacerations, broken bones or worse. Their safety depends on you and your ability to pay attention and keep a safe environment for the elderly person.

Depending upon the stage of the disease, various aspects of an Alzheimer's patient's disease can get in the way of their safety. These include:

- **A lack of judgment**: He or she can forget how to make use of ordinary household appliances.

- **Losing a sense of time and place**: He or she can walk on their own street and can get lost even though they've lived there a long time.

- **Behavioral issues**: Increasing confusion, suspiciousness and fear are likely to lead to unexpected behaviors.

- **Changes in physical ability**: Balance problems can lead to trips and falls in or outside the home.

- **Sensory changes**: There will be visual misperception, changes in hearing, differing sensitivity to temperature and poor depth perception.

The trick is to take proper precautions so you can improve safety and make sure injuries don't happen to your loved one with dementia. The better your safety measures, the longer your loved one can remain independent or at least not living in a nursing facility.

Safety in Home

Depending on how far into the dementia the person is, safety measures can be put into place so that the dementia patient can live independently or in the caregivers home for a long time. The person's abilities will change over time so ongoing creativity may be necessary to keep them living safely in a home environment.

It pays to evaluate your environment to see which areas are at the highest risk. Remove things that can be harmful and find creative ways to keep the dementia patient as far away from dangerous rooms and areas as possible. Even substances can be dangerous, not unlike living with a toddler. Basic household objects can be dangerous things to an elderly dementia patient. Make sure you keep these items away from your loved one. Try to make use of appliances that have an automatic shut-off feature. Keep your loved one away from any type of water source.

Put a circuit breaker or a hidden gas valve on the stove and oven so that the elderly person can't accidentally turn these things on. You can also take the knobs off the burners so that only those with access to the knobs can turn on the stove elements. Keep lawn mowers, grills, power tools, cleaning products and knives away from anyone who doesn't have the judgment to use them. Get rid of toxic plants and certain decorative fruits that can accidentally be eaten as regular food.

Put prescription drugs, vitamins, fake sugar and seasonings in a lock box of some kind that is difficult to get into. Supervise the use of alcohol and tobacco by the dementia patient. These can interact with their medications and can have bad side effects.

If you have a firearm in the house, there are special precautions you need to take. Lock up all firearms in a locked cabinet or storage case and keep the ammunition in a different location, also locked. Keep firearms completely unloaded when stored in the house. If you want to get rid of a weapon, ask for help from law enforcement.

Most of the major injuries and accidents happen when the elderly person is doing normal daily activities like using the restroom, bathing and eating. For this reason, you need to check the temperature of all water and food sources because the elderly person can't always tell the difference between things that are hot or cold. Put in a walk-in shower that has grab bars for balance and safety. Put textured stickers on slippery surfaces. If you have rugs, put adhesives under them so they don't move. Better yet, remove all slippery rugs altogether.

Remember that color differentiation is difficult in elderly dementia patients and differences in levels of light can confuse and disorient the individual. Make sure that entries, landings and things like stairways and bathrooms are well lit with extra lighting. Hallways, bathrooms and bedrooms should be equipped with nightlights.

Have doctors' names and contact information readily available along with a list of medications the patient is taking, including times and dosages. Make a list of allergies to drugs and foods. Keep these along with legal papers, such as the person's advanced directives, living will and power of attorney. Put down contact information of family and friends to call in case of an emergency. Health insurance information is very important to have on hand as well. Put all of these documents for when the dementia patient is hospitalized or when you travel. Have copies of these documents stored somewhere away from your home.

Wandering Behaviors

The patient with dementia is at great risk for wandering, even in the neighborhood, and getting lost. Many do this as a regular behavior. More that 60 percent of dementia patients will have wandering behaviors and if not found within a 24 hour period of time, half of them will be dead or will have suffered serious injury.

Signs of wandering behavior include coming back from a routine walk at a time that is later than expected. If they try to go to work when they no longer work, they are at risk. They are also at risk when they attempt to go "home" when they are already there or if they are restless, pacing or undergoing repetitive behaviors. If the person can't find their own bedroom or bathroom, they may wander to try and find them. Patients who act out chores or hobbies but don't actually get anything accomplished, they are at risk for wandering behavior. If they become anxious in crowded conditions, they are possibly a wandering risk.

You can reduce wandering behavior by providing the dementia patient with structured and meaningful activities they easily know how to do. Allow the patient to get enough healthy exercise, which helps decrease anxiety, restlessness and agitation. Put dead-bolts on exterior doors that are either really high or really low. Make sure that you keep up with toileting, thirst and hunger so they aren't agitated because of these reasons. Try to be reassuring when the patient feels lost, disoriented or abandoned. Make sure the access to the car keys is limited. Stay away from crowded places that can confuse and disorient the individual (like shopping malls). Don't leave the dementia patient alone, especially in unfamiliar surroundings.

When a Dementia Patient Drives

The act of driving requires that the driver have good judgment, fast reaction times and quick decision making. Because Alzheimer's disease is so progressive, they will go from being a driving person to being one that does not drive. Talk to your loved ones about when the time will come that the person can no longer drive an automobile. The transition can be made easier by having a specific plan in place as to what to do when driving is no longer possible.

The following are signs that it is time to quit driving include:

- Failing to observe traffic signs

- Forgetting how to find their way to familiar spots

- Slow decision making

- Poor decision making

- Traveling at inappropriate speeds

- Hitting curbs while driving

- Becoming confused and angry while driving

- Crossing lanes inappropriately

- Making mistakes at intersections

- Mixing up the brake pedal and the accelerator

- Returning home later than expected

When the dementia patient loses the ability to drive, he or she can be very upset. If the person doesn't understand and insists on driving past the point in time when driving is safe, friends and family members need to pull together and think about other options. This might involve having the doctor write a "do not drive" prescription for the patient or having law enforcement give the dementia patient a ticket or citation. You can hide the automobile keys and disable the car in some way so it won't run. Keep the car out of eye sight so the patient isn't reminded of it. When in doubt, have the dementia patient evaluated by the Department of Safety or the Department of Motor Vehicles.

Traveling Safely

There may come a time that you'll wish to travel with your loved one who also happens to have dementia. You can have an enjoyable and safe trip if you follow certain tips and understand that the level of confusion will necessarily go up when you bring your loved one into unfamiliar circumstances.

Make sure you pack all important health documents, including lists of medications, dosages and living will, among other things. Make sure the elderly person had comfortable clothing to change into and safe walking shoes. Pack snacks for everyone and have activities for the elderly person to do.

Travel to known and familiar destinations and make sure the daily routine doesn't get very much disrupted. Inform the staff of the hotel you are staying in about any special needs you have. Do your traveling when things are usually good with the dementia patient. The local Alzheimer's Association office at your destination may be of help.

Going on an airplane takes special precautions. The whole milieu of the place can be distracting or overwhelming to the Alzheimer's patient. Inform the airport medical service that you will be traveling through the airport. You may wish to use a wheelchair or other services. Let the in-flight crew know of your special needs.

In Preparation for a Disaster

Floods, forest fires or hurricanes can happen in any locale and it can be upsetting for everyone. Preparing for these events can make things as safe as possible in case of these kinds of emergencies.

Think about an emergency kit you have pulled together in preparation for a disaster. This kit should have all the important documents as listed above pulled together. It should contain several changes of clothing, extra medication, incontinence products (if needed), a Medic Alert device, an ID bracelet, a recent picture of the dementia patient, favorite items of food and bottled water for the Alzheimer's patient.

Make sure you keep in mind that your loved one may need to escape a disaster situation in a wheelchair or with the use of a cane. They may not move quickly in the event of a disaster. If your loved one lives in a nursing home, find out what their disaster plan and evacuation plan are. Most should be able to give you a written disaster plan that you should know about.

Summary

Safety is vitally important in the care of a patient with dementia. They have limitations in judgment, balance, vision and other abilities so that caring for them can be difficult and sometimes dangerous. One needs to take a close look at the hazards in the home and change them so that the elderly person has no access to pills, poisons, firearms or things they can fall down. It means putting locks on doors, hiding items you don't want the person to become involved with and pulling up throw rugs that can trip up the dementia patient.

This is an individual who will begin their disease as a driving person but will one day become unable to safely drive. A plan needs to come into play so as to make the transition from driving to not driving as smooth as possible.

Accidents and injuries are major causes of death in the Alzheimer's patient. As a caregiver, it is important to keep an eye out on the Alzheimer's loved one just as you would a toddler. With proper care and attention to detail, you can care for a loved one with Alzheimer's dementia who lives injury free.

Chapter 4: Caregivers for Alzheimer's Disease Patients

Unpaid Caregivers

There are more than 15 million unpaid caregivers of patients with Alzheimer's disease in the US today. These are family members, neighbors, friends and members of the person's church who together work to keep the Alzheimer's patient out of the nursing home as long as possible. These people put in 17.4 billion hours of unpaid care at an annual cost of more than $210 billion USD.

Eighty percent of all dementia care is given by family members. Only about ten percent of Alzheimer's adults receive the entirety of their care by paid care workers. This care of Alzheimer's patients is extremely difficult, resulting in emotional stress and depression on the part of the unpaid worker. This kind of work can have a bad impact on the employment status, financial picture, health and personal relationships of the caregiver. There needs to be as much in place as possible to help caregivers do the job they do.

There is a survey done every year to understand just who the caregivers are for these kinds of patients. It's called the Behavioral Risk Factor Surveillance System or BRFSS survey and it's an annual telephone survey done with the help of the US Centers for Disease Control and Prevention. A recent survey showed that dementia caregivers tend to be older than caregivers of other kinds of people. They tended to be female and Caucasian.

The Alzheimer's Association came up with these data on the demographics of Alzheimer's caregivers:

- Under age 35: 10 percent

- 35-44: 11 percent

- 45-54: 23 percent

- 55-64: 33 percent

- 65-84: 21 percent

- 85 years and older: 2 percent

Most caregivers were aged 55 and older and most do not have a college education. They are usually the primary breadwinners of the household with nearly half of the caregivers being employed at least part time. Half of all caregivers lived within the same household as the Alzheimer's patient. Thirty percent were also caring for children who were under the age of 18 at the same time. Some people refer to these caregivers as the "sandwich generation" — asked to care for people younger in age and older in age than they are. Almost half of all caregivers are caring for their parents and many are taking care of their children.

Around 6-17 percent are caring for a spouse. Nine percent of caregivers unfortunately live at least two hours away from the person they are tending to and about 6 percent live between one and two hours distance away from the person whose care depends on them. This means that between 1.4 million and 2.3 million caregivers of Alzheimer's patients can be considered long distance care givers and this can prove to be quite dangerous.

There are some ethnic differences in dementia caregivers. Those who were non-Hispanic whites were about 70-81 percent of the total, while African Americans made up 8 percent. Hispanics amounted to between 1 and 12 percent of the total number of caregivers. Asians accounted for 1-2 percent of the total. It's difficult to compare the different characteristics of caregivers because there are so few non-white caregivers.

Some differences noted were that Caucasians (non-Hispanic) are more likely to care for an Alzheimer's parent at 54 percent when compared to non-whites (38 percent. Asians living in America and whites are more likely to care for a married person when compared to African American caregivers. Hispanic and African-American caregivers spent more time in caregiving (up to 30 hours per week) than White caregivers (around 19.8 hours per week). Those who spent more time caring for their loved one had a higher emotional burden than those who spent less time caregiving.

What are the main tasks you might do in caring for a loved one who has Alzheimer's disease?

- You might be instrumental in activities of daily living like cooking, dressing, bathing and hygiene.

- You might shop for groceries, prepare meals or provide transportation for doctors' appointments.

- You can help the person take their medications properly and follow doctor's orders

- You can manage legal affairs and finances.

- You can help them with personal activities of daily living.

- You can help them with grooming, dressing, bathing, feeding and toileting

- You can be the manager of the person's behavioral issues and safety problems

- You can assist in transferring and with mobility

- You can supervise the individual when doing unsafe activities

- You might be called upon to find supportive services for when you're gone

- You can arrange for medical care and doctor's appointments

- You might hire and supervise paid workers.

- You will perform household cleaning and chores.

- You will deal with family members regarding communication about the patient

More than 50 percent of all unpaid caregivers are responsible for getting the patient in and out of bed. A third of all caregivers help their loved one get on and off the toilet, managing incontinence issues, bathing and feeding the Alzheimer's patient. This is not much of an issue if the parent or patient doesn't have dementia.

Almost 2/3 of all unpaid caregivers are advocates for their loved ones when it comes to service providers and government agencies. Nearly half supervise the paid caregivers from government or other agencies. When the patient with Alzheimer's disease moves to an assisted living facility or nursing home, the job of the unpaid caregiver usually changes. They still assist with financial recordkeeping and legal issues, make doctors' appointments and provide important emotional support. Sometimes there is still a need for an unpaid caregiver to help with dressing, bathing and hygiene.

It turns out that the duration of care when the person has Alzheimer's disease is longer than if the person is elderly but doesn't have Alzheimer's disease. A total of 43 percent of people had been caregivers for 1-4 years, according to one study and 32 percent had been caregivers for five years or longer.

In 2011, the fifteen million unpaid caregivers of those with Alzheimer's disease provided a total of 17.4 billion USD in care at an average of 21.9 hours of unpaid care provided per week or about 1,140 hours of care per year. The estimate pay for these people were they paid workers was $12.12 per hour. This amounts to $210 billion USD in care provided by unpaid caregivers in the US for Alzheimer's patients.

Things that increase the amount of care an unpaid caregiver provides to a loved one include living with the loved one, having the disease progress to becoming severe and having the dementia patient suffer from another coexisting medical condition such as heart disease, stroke or cancer.

There are many challenges to caring for a loved one with Alzheimer's disease. This can include difficulty related to memory loss. The dementia patient can fail to remember the caregiver or can fail to remember appointments or activities that may already have taken place. The patient has sensory deficits and communication deficits which make it difficult for communication to take place. They have poor judgment and can be quite oppositional at times. As the person needs an increased amount of personal care, there can be increased opposition to that type of care. They may object to supervision and be wandering throughout the house and out of the house.

These are the times that the caregiver undergoes a great deal of stress. The relationship between the caregiver and their loved one is changing and the personality changes/oppositional behavior can be very stressful. Because the relationship between the caregiver and elderly person has been so close over the years, the caregiver can see these changes in their loved one and can suffer from psychological or physical illnesses themselves.

Even though caregivers often feel positive feelings about the job they do helping their elderly loved one and focus on family togetherness and personal satisfaction, they still are dealing with stress regarding the care they give. For example:

Sixty one percent of unpaid caregivers of dementia patients rate their stress level as high or very high and 33 percent of these people report feeling somewhat depressed. Many report a great deal of "caregiving strain" regarding their financial issues and their other family relationships. When compared to people who took care of those who didn't have dementia, 36.5 percent of Alzheimer's caregivers said that stress was their greatest problem. This was the case in only 23.6 percent of people who cared for those that didn't have dementia.

Caregivers often have to change their working hours, take a demotion to care for their loved one, give up their jobs altogether or retire early because they don't have the time or opportunity to care for their loved one in the way it needs to happen. Some attempted to work but were fired due to poor performance.

A survey by the NAC and AARP found that 40 percent of all Alzheimer's caregivers reported having a high degree of emotional distress. These were people who were often female and were the primary caregiver who lived with the recipient of the care. They often felt they had no choice in becoming the caregiver. When the behavioral symptoms get too severe, the stress only gets worse and there is an increased likelihood of putting their loved one in a nursing home. Even after placement, however, there is an increase in stress above baseline.

When it comes to placement in a nursing home, most agree there is no right or wrong time to make the placement. When stress levels get too high or it becomes unsafe to have the individual remain in the home, placing them in a nursing home may be the only real option.

The care gets really intense in the last year of the dementia patient's life. In this period of time, the caregiver is on duty 24 hours per day and 7 days a week. This is a time that is really distressful—so stressful that 72 percent of caregivers felt relief when their loved ones died.

Caregivers become secondary patients, in part because of the negative impact caring for another person has on their health. They can suffer from psychological illnesses, an increase in chronic illnesses and even death. They may find themselves seeing the doctor more often for diseases they wouldn't have had if they weren't Alzheimer's caregivers. Stress has been reported as very high or high about 43 percent of the time. There are about $8.7 billion USD added to the US healthcare costs because of care given to caregivers.

Caregivers find themselves to be very concerned about their own health at a rate of 75 percent because they need to be healthy to be a good caregiver. On the other hand, caregivers were more likely than those who did not give care to another to have health they rated fair or poor. They were more likely to say that giving care to the Alzheimer's patient made their health more poorly. They were more likely to believe that the act of caregiving was the main thing that exacerbated their ill health.

Even though caregivers are less likely to exercise than non-caregivers, the caregivers do get exercise just by caring for their loved ones. Getting them bathed or in an out of bed takes energy and exercise. Some research is suggesting that caregivers are at risk for a condition called metabolic syndrome. This is a combination of high blood pressure, truncal obesity, diabetes, high triglycerides and heart disease. They also have higher levels of stress hormones, poor immune function, increased incidence of high blood pressure, slow wound healing and an increased risk of cardiac disease, even without metabolic syndrome.

The health of the dementia patient can have a negative impact on the health of the caregiver. Caregivers of a person with dementia when the dementia patient is hospitalized are much more likely to die in the year following the hospitalization when compared to caregivers of the elderly who didn't have dementia and was hospitalized.

A total of 44 percent of the caregivers of the dementia patient were employed at least part time, although 65 percent had to take time off because of their caregiving duties. Twenty percent had to take leaves of absence because of the need to care for a loved one with dementia.

Unpaid caregivers are necessary parts of what it takes to see that a person with Alzheimer's disease is able to stay at home and avoid the intensive costs of nursing home care. An unpaid caregiver is usually the spouse, child or niece/nephew of the dementia patient and is often put under a great deal of financial stress, emotional stress and physical stress. This is why paid caregivers are sometimes hired.

Paid Caregivers

There are many paid caregivers of Alzheimer's persons. These include direct care workers such as home health aides, nurse's aides, personal aides and home care aides. They receive special training in the care of elderly people and take advice and direction from doctors, physician's assistants, nurses and social workers.

Direct care workers do many things for the elderly person including dressing, bathing, food preparation, feeding and housekeeping. Some stay round the clock and aid in toileting. They directly influence the care of these elderly workers and have jobs that are both rewarding and challenging.

The training they receive includes programming in diseases of the elderly, behavioral techniques with regard to the Alzheimer's patient, personal cares, nutrition and issues around cognitive impairment in Alzheimer's patients.

Experts believe that the US will need an additional 3.5 million health care workers by the year 2030 to meet the demand of extra Alzheimer's disease patients. Unfortunately, few providers have decided to choose this path. The pay is not really great and there is training involved in becoming a health care provider. The work is also very difficult and in some cases, is not all that rewarding. There are even very few doctors involved in geriatric medicine—only about 7000 geriatric medicine doctors certified per year. Only about 1600 geriatric psychiatry specialists were certified per year. By the year 2030, it is estimated that 36,000 geriatric specialists will be needed to meet the demands of the population at that time.

In other specialties, there are also low numbers helping the elderly. For example, only 1 percent of registered nurses, 1 percent of physician assistants, 1 percent of pharmacists and 4 percent of social workers actually profess to work specifically with the elderly.

Summary

Unpaid caregivers of patients with Alzheimer's disease are often unaffected spouses, children, grandchildren and other relatives or friends who have dedicated their lives to caring for difficult patients with Alzheimer's disease.

This is a very difficult task to take up and there is often a lot of stress put on the part of the caregiver who must deal with the risk of accidents, health issues and behavioral issues of their elderly loved one. Many live in the same home as the person they are caring for so they can help with bathing, dressing, meal preparation and toileting.

Over time, the Alzheimer's patient gets worse and the stress on the caregiver only gets greater. At some point the patient dies or requires so much care that they are transferred over to the nursing home for extended care.

Some families can afford paid care by a nurse's assistant or home health care worker to take care of the Alzheimer's patient on a periodic basis for respite care or for more longstanding care, especially when the patient lives with a spouse who can do some things but can't do things like bathing or dressing the patient. This is where a nursing assistant or other paid worker can come in handy and can offset care given by family members.

Chapter 5: Feeding and Nutrition in Alzheimer's Disease

People with Alzheimer's disease often have difficulty eating. Swallowing becomes difficult in the late stages of the disease and many have problems getting the food onto the spoon or fork and into the mouth. Foods can taste different to them from their pre-disease state and they can have problems with dentures and eating hard foods. It is up to the caregiver to prepare a meal for the elderly person that is easy to eat, nutritious and promotes healthy weight gain. Many with Alzheimer's disease lose weight because they don't get enough calories in their body.

There is no "special diet" required for those who have Alzheimer's dementia unless they have high blood pressure or perhaps diabetes—both of which need dietary changes. Instead, they need a well-balanced, healthy diet containing a variety of foods from each food group.

Keep track of the rough amount of calories taken in by the Alzheimer's patient. It should be about 2000 calories or more per day. Too many days of less than this and you will see weight loss that is difficult to gain back. Chronic weight loss affects the body's immune system and the skin often becomes devoid of fat, and papery or thin. Malnourished bodies get more cuts and bruises because they lack fat protection in the tissues.

Make sure you cut down on cholesterol, saturated fats and sugars. The elderly are just as prone to getting blockages of the arteries or diabetes so the diet should reflect those possibilities. There is plenty to eat without eating saturated fat, cholesterol or added sugar. Limit the amount of sodium in food preparation and don't use table salt when eating. This can only bring up the blood pressure on the elderly person, who usually has stiff arteries that are more prone to fluctuations in blood pressure. Unless the individual has a fluid restriction because of congestive heart failure or liver disease, water should be plentiful to keep the elderly person hydrated. Keep track of how much they urinate and if they don't urinate within 4-6 hours during the day, they are probably not getting enough.

Make sure you find out from the doctor whether or not any foods interfere with medications the elderly person is taking. Your doctor may be able to change some medications to cut down on any food-related side effects so the person can eat a more well-rounded diet.

Constipation is a big problem among the elderly, especially if they are not very physically active. The trick is to eat plenty of fruits, vegetables, and foods containing whole grains. Each of these food groups are excellent sources of fiber, which can combat constipation. Also remember that plenty of fluids keep constipation away as well. Remain as physically active as possible.

Food is difficult to eat when you suffer from dry mouth. Dry mouth is caused by mouth breathing, dehydration and is a natural phenomenon of old age. Food is difficult to swallow when you have dry mouth. The signal for thirst is lessened with Alzheimer's disease so they are more likely to get a dry mouth than other elderly people. You can try to dunk hard foods like bread, crackers or cookies in coffee, hot chocolate or milk to soften them before eating. Take a drink of water between bites of food. Add gravies or broth to foods to soften them up. Eat candy that is sour or chew on fruit ice to increase the amount of saliva you make and to moisten your mouth.

Malnutrition, as mentioned, is a big problem with the Alzheimer's patient. They often suffer from poor nutrition and have difficulties swallowing and eating healthy foods. They sometimes can't self-feed and make poor choices in foods they eat. Depression can affect the amount of food they take in.

In order to try to combat weight loss and nutrition, you need to attempt to have the person eat several small meals per day up to 6 times daily. This keeps them full and eating on a regular basis. Have them take a multivitamin with mineral supplement. Eat the food that is more nutritious earlier in the meal and prepare foods that are easier to eat. Have them eat with others so as to make the eating experience as pleasant as possible.

Talk to the doctor if you need help around eating or swallowing. He or she can order a swallow study to see which foods or liquids are having problems going down. This can help you change the diet so as to avoid choking. Some foods are easier to swallow than others.

Maintain the best oral hygiene as possible. Brush and floss the teeth of the elderly person and clean the dentures daily. Make sure the dentures fit and make sure you make regular dental appointments for the elderly person. Routine cleanings are a must.

Be careful with the type of utensils you use. You may need to resort to using spoons and bowls to serve food rather than plates and forks. Cut up food into bite sized pieces so that the individual can just spoon pieces of food into his or her mouth. Finger foods are also good options for feeding the patient with Alzheimer's disease. If the person remains physically active, they will be hungrier than if they are inactive. If they are depressed, they may not have a good appetite. Talk to your doctor if you think you need to make any specific dietary changes in your elderly person's diet. A nutritionist may actually be helpful.

How to Make Eating Pleasurable

There are ways to enhance the meal experience that can improve the quality and quantity of eating for the person with Alzheimer's disease. You can set the table neatly and nicely, using napkins and placemats. Try different colors on different days. Keep distracting things off the table while eating.

Make sure the table is of the right height and accommodates a wheelchair if necessary. Keep music to a minimum as this can be agitating to the eater. Soft classical music can be a perfect choice. Make sure the room itself is not too busy so the person can focus on eating and only eating. Keep busy wall decorations off the walls and make the room well lit so they can see their food. If not using a wheelchair, use a chair that has good back support.

Choose food cutlery that can be held easily and that are not dangerous. Have big napkins to catch food that drops and to wipe up the food afterward. Put the food directly on the plate or in the bowl and keep serving dishes (which can be distracting) off the table. Scent the area with vanilla or mint to stimulate the senses and the appetite.

Try to eat all together in a family environment. This will stimulate eating and the person will feel better eating with others. It can revive memories about eating as a family. So, turn the TV off and have the meal already at the table before calling the elderly person to the table.

How to Make Food Fun and Easy to Eat

There are things you can do to help keep food safe and yet tasty to eat. Swallowing is a difficulty in Alzheimer's persons so you need to make food that is easy to swallow and easy to get from the dish to the mouth.

Select soft foods like soups or puddings that don't really need to be chewed and instead can be easily swallowed. These foods can taste good and can be just as flavorful as hard food. Look for a recipe book specifically designed for making soft foods. Make sure you know first aid around choking issues in case something does happen. Make sure they sit up before and following the meal so that food keeps going down smoothly. Make sure you give plenty of reminders to the person to keep swallowing.

To prevent choking, moisten the food with sauces or gravy to make it moist enough to go down without pain. Thicken liquids, which are easy to choke on. They make thickening powders that can reduce ability of the liquid to slip down the trachea where it doesn't belong. Add mashed potato flakes, corn starch or flour to some liquids to keep them from being too fluid.

Mash, chop, or puree foods in a food processor or blender because it won't have to be chewed much to get down. Have them tuck the chin down when swallowing to promote a healthy swallow. You can gently stroke the person's throat to promote swallowing.

Try to make finger foods like small sandwiches, slices of fruits and sandwiches with buns. These are easier to hold and to chew than other foods. Make as many handheld foods as possible.

Teach the elderly person to eat slowly so that eating slowly can be automatic. Find special utensils designed for people with poor grip strengths. Simple dishes like soups and stews are easy to eat and can be made thick enough to be safe to swallow. Use non-spill cups for liquids. You can even serve soup in one of these cups. Brightly colored plates, bowls and cups can make the food on these dishes more appetizing. Use a wet cloth and place it beneath eating dishes to keep the dishes from sliding around.

Summary

Food and eating are important daily events in the life of the person with dementia. As a caregiver, you need to make sure your loved one is eating enough because if they lose weight, it will be very difficult to gain it back. Things like swallowing and choking are important issues and food can be created that doesn't cause swallowing or choking problems.

The diet should be as balanced as possible with fruit, vegetables, whole grains and dairy products. The food should be as flavorful as possible because the elderly patient can't taste things as strongly as younger people. You need to make sure the temperature of the food is safely not too hot and not too cold. Their sense of hot and cold is diminished as we age.

Make sure the environment around eating is as friendly as possible but without the distractions that can make it difficult for the individual to eat without becoming agitated.

Chapter 6: Behavior Problems in the Elderly

Behavioral problems are one of the most vexing things a caregiver has to deal with. It is estimated that between 80 percent and 90 percent of patients with dementia will develop at least one problematic behavioral symptom while having their illness.

One common way to describe this type of behavior is "agitation", which involves inappropriate vocal, verbal or motor activity that is not seen by an outside person to result from a specific need.

Four kinds of agitated behavior can be described:

1. Verbal nonaggressive behavior like negativism and complaining

2. Verbal aggressive behavior such as screaming behaviors, making

strange noises, cursing, verbal sexual advances

3. Physical nonaggressive, such as performing repetitive behavior, inappropriately dressing, disrobing and eating inappropriate substances. It can also mean a general restlessness, moving furniture around and hiding things or hoarding things.

4. Physical aggressiveness, which means sexual advances, hurting oneself or others, and throwing things. It can involve pushing, pulling hair, kicking, scratching, hitting and biting.

In reality, people with dementia begin to lose their "inner critic" which would normally tell them if something is inappropriate or not. The dementia patient may curse a lot and may consume alcohol more than they did when not suffering from dementia. They utter basic expressions that many of us think about but do not shout out like dementia patients do. When the patient with dementia is frustrated or surprised, he or she may have curse words pop up in their head and on their lips.

They also seem to forget socially appropriate norms. They may shoplift or take off their clothes in front of visitors. Sexual nuances or behaviors are common. The sexual behavior can be toward those they know or toward complete strangers.

Caregivers need to learn how to be firm and respectful toward the elderly dementia patient. Things like refocusing them on other activities are perfect ways to stop abnormal behavior. Caregivers should avoid getting angry with the dementia patient because they usually do not understand what it is they are doing. In the late stages of dementia, the person is often overstimulated, frustrated by changes in routine and possibly suffering from physical discomfort and becomes agitate because they don't know how to communicate or express themselves.

Medications for Behavioral Issues

Certain medications, such as memantine and cholinesterase inhibitors, slow the progression of the dementia, especially in the early stages. They are also used to control problem behaviors that result from having dementia.

Anxiolytic medication helps control the fear and agitation that comes from not being comfortable in strange surroundings and being incapable of controlling a chaotic environment they live in. In early dementia, you can teach them relaxation techniques, exercise and meditative techniques that help avoid outbursts of emotions and panic attacks.

Commonly used drugs for anxiety include:

- Buspar (buspirone)

- Ativan (lorazepam)

- Klonopin (clonazepam)

- Xanax (alprazolam)

- Valium (diazepam)

- Serax (oxazepam)

Medications for Depression

Many dementia patients suffer from depression. If you think about it, they have lost their independence, their mobility and have fewer interactions with the world around them. This can cause a poor appetite, tiredness and reduced interest in activities of daily living. They can use any one of a number of antidepressants can improve the patient's mood and their ability to function. Some commonly used antidepressants in the elderly include:

- Celexa (citalopram)

- Paxil (paroxetine)

- Effexor (venlafaxine)

- Prozac (fluoxetine)

- Zoloft (sertraline)

The Use of Antipsychotics

Antipsychotics help the Alzheimer's patient get back the difference between reality and fantasy. Without the help of these medications, there can be paranoid ideation, hallucination and elaborate delusions. In these types of cases, anxiolytic medication alone may not be enough to make the dementia patient feel better and behave better. Commonly used drugs include the following:

- Clozaril (clozapine)

- Abilify (aripiprazole)

- Geodon (ziprasidone)

- Risperdal (risperidone)

- Zyprexa (olanzepine)

- Seroquel (quetiapine)

Hypnotic Medication

Sleep difficulties are common in patients with Alzheimer's disease. Yet too many medications used in younger people will be too much for the elderly patient and they can be tired during the day as well. In order to decrease daytime napping, medications to help the person sleep better can be used that are fairly short acting and do not cause daytime sleepiness. These medications include:

- Ambien (zolpidem)

- Sonata (zaleplon)

- Restoril (temazepam)

The idea behind these types of medication is to make sure the dementia person and the caregiver is safe and that the dementia patient feels better. There are many behavioral techniques that can be used to avoid medication but if these don't work, the medications may have to be tried. Some forms of dementia do not respond as well to these drugs than others. Talk to your loved one's doctor about what medications might be helpful and what suggestions they have for keeping uncomfortable behaviors at bay without medications. Pay attention to side effects which would necessitate stopping the medication, such as fatigue and balance difficulties

Behavioral Suggestions for the Caregiver

Let's take a look at some specific problem behaviors that come up when caring for Alzheimer's disease patients:

- **When the person refuses help**. The person might refuse help from anyone or just accept help from one person. In such cases, consider your approach. If they don't want help, consider having them work on their own at the task for a while before coming back and asking them again. Give them plenty of warning in advance of an event that might be upsetting, like having toenails clipped or getting a haircut. Sometimes it helps to give them a task to do while you're doing another task. For example, you could ask them to comb their hair while you get their socks and shoes on. It gives them a sense of independence and yet gets things done at the same time.

- **When there is hoarding behavior**. People with Alzheimer's disease tend to form collections of things like food that helps them feel safe and in control. Hiding places tend to be drawers or beneath beds and mattresses. It is a good idea to go through the garbage or through dirty laundry. Keep some cabinets locked in order to keep them clean and organized. Try not to confront their bad behavior as most of the time, it is benign and won't hurt anyone.

- **Repetitive behaviors**. Dementia patients often ask the same things over and over again or do the same things over and over again. They can even pace back and forth. You might have to simply accept the behavior as it is usually harmless. You can redirect the behavior by having them do something else.

- **Lack of sleep**. Dementia suffers often have difficulty sleeping. They may sleep all day but be up throughout the night. Try to use artificial lighting or open the draperies to give cues to the loved one that it is daytime. Use these same cues to make sure they know it is dark time and time to sleep. Keep the person up during the day if possible and avoid giving them caffeine after lunch. Try engaging them in simple exercises or in activities they can do during the day so that they are tired enough to sleep. If all else fails, try a medication that promotes sleep. Talk to your doctor about getting a prescription. Remember that it is dangerous to have a dementia patient awake and wandering when you are sleeping.

- **Sundowning behavior**. This is when the patient with dementia suffers from an increase in disorientation, agitation, confusion and other behaviors that start at sundown and last into the night. It is possibly due to fatigue or with problems in the patient's biological clock. You can eliminate some of the symptoms of sundowning by closing the drapes and turning on inside lighting so they can't tell it's nighttime. If sleepless and behaviors persist, see the doctor about prescribing a medication that can act as a hypnotic for sleeping.

- **Wandering behaviors**. It is estimated that 60 percent of people with Alzheimer's dementia will wander away from their home and get lost. The individual with the disease loses the memory of where they live and what the location looks like. Simple forgetfulness can become dangerous when the person actually leaves home and walks away.

Reasons for wandering behavior can include: having too much energy; being bored with one's surroundings; trying to walk off muscle discomfort and the belief that the loved one has to go somewhere.

It helps to try to understand exactly why wandering occurs in your situation so you can think of more appropriate responses. You can, for example, tray to go on more walks with the loved ones to tire them out and to decrease wandering.

Make sure the loved one wears some kind of identification on them at all times. It can be an ID bracelet or necklace—anything that doesn't come off easily. You can get such products from Safe Return or Project Lifesaver that will provide you with ID information and medical information. Your address and phone number can be included. There is also an Alzheimer's Association Safe Return Program and other programs in the community that can help find and return an Alzheimer's patient.

Try to install locks on the external doors of your home that are near the top or bottom of the doorway. It is safe because others can get out the door in an emergency but the Alzheimer's patient usually can't find or figure out the lock. Caregivers can also set up a fenced-in yard. Be sure to have a current photo of your loved one for police or searchers to use in order to find the lost person.

- **Hallucinations and delusions**. Dementia can change how a person sees the world and they will often hear or see things that aren't there. In the early stages of the disease, the person will recognize that what they are perceiving is a figment of their imagination. As the disease gets worse, however, they won't be able to distinguish reality from fantasy and can act out their hallucinations and delusions, unable to be swayed that they aren't true.

Hallucinations can involve imaginary smells, feelings, visual cues, tastes, or auditory cues. They are the result of damage to the brain and chemical changes in the brain that cause sensory changes made worse in the presence of fatigue, infections or nutritional deficits.

Delusions are false beliefs or understandings about what is going on in the present time. It could become a belief that the person is being poisoned or that people are stealing things from the person. Delusional behavior can be very hard to deal with because the dementia patient isn't trusting of anyone, including their caregivers. Medications like atypical antipsychotics can be used to prevent these kinds of phenomena.

Speak to the doctor about possible reasons behind delusional behavior or hallucinations. They can be due to fatigue and there may need to be a change in the way the dementia patient sleeps. If the person is not harming themselves or others, you might want to reason with the Alzheimer's patient or just ignore minor hallucinations.

Try the 3 R's, which are **Reassurance, Refocusing and Responding**. When there is anger and emotional reactions to hallucinations, respond to their fears and try different tactics to get them distracted from the emotionality of the experience. Acknowledge their experience but give them a lesson in reality at the same time.

Try and think about why the person is having a delusion or hallucination at that moment. Does the situation remind the elderly person of something in their past? Is there something chaotic going on that is adversely affecting the environment of the individual? Keep a journal or record about when and where the person experiences the most hallucinations and what is going on at that time. What events are happening at the time that might be triggering the person to hallucinate? Do what you can to calm the individual's anxiety and fear.

Address the issue as it is happening. Create some kind of activity that refocuses the attention of the person with dementia who is hallucinating or having delusions. Make sure the room is well lit and without a lot of distractions. Even simple things like televisions and radios can turn into objects triggering auditory or visual hallucinations. Covering the windows with shades can diminish the delusion that someone is being watched.

- **Driving can become both dangerous and risky** when the dementia patient gets behind the wheel. The hardest decision a family and Alzheimer's patient must make is when to stop driving and often the Alzheimer's patient is resistant to stopping driving. It is often the focus in the family of controversy or frustration.

When a loved one loses the ability to drive, it means a big loss of independence and a lack of control. The person cannot move around independently and can't go places. Even so, safety takes precedence and the right decision must be made around whether or not the person can drive.

Driving is actually quite a complex task that cannot usually be done by the moderately affected patient. The driver must be able to recognize the meaning of traffic signs, know the meaning of traffic signals, pay attention to the existence of other cars, react to the movement of other cars, adapt their driving skills to the weather or road changes and handle other details of driving cars such as knowing the difference between the brake pedal and the accelerator.

There are signs to look out for that will tell you that your loved one is not ready to drive. For example, if the person with dementia becomes confused, frustrated or angry while driving or if the caregiver has concerns about the loved one's reaction times, visual limitations or hearing limitations, there may be reason to stop driving. If the Alzheimer's patient doesn't obey or even notice traffic signs or isn't using proper driving etiquette, this may be the time to quit driving.

It actually pays to plan ahead when the Alzheimer's patient has mild disease. It pays to have a discussion over what kind of situation should stop the person from driving. If this can't be done, it is up to the caregiver to make the decision as to when the person should stop driving. Try to honestly address your concerns to see if you can convince the person to quit driving. If you can't, try to get a recommendation from the family lawyer or family doctor. If all else fails, hide the keys or get rid of the car.

There are other options for transportation that the Alzheimer's patient can use while they are still mobile. They can use the bus or perhaps use community transportation services that help the elderly get to the store or to doctors' appointments. If travel is impossible, think about having things like groceries and medications delivered to the home.

Why Do Dementia Patients Get Behavioral Problems?

There are many theories around why behavioral problems are so common in the dementia patient. There is, for example, the direct impact model, which says that there are organically deteriorated parts of the brain and pathophysiological damage that directly result in changes in behavior.

There is the Unmet Needs Model that says dementia causes a decrease in the ability to have one's needs met due to a limited ability to communicate. The needs can be physical, environmental, emotional or social. These needs can include relief of pain or other physical discomfort, mental issues like anxiety and depression, an uncomfortable environment, a lack of proper social contacts, or stimulation that is either too little or too much.

There is the Behavioral Model which believes that problem behaviors are controlled by its antecedents and consequences. They learn behaviors that are reinforced by staff members or family members. If, for example, the agitated person gets extra attention, this might precipitate more activity of a similar nature.

There is also the Environmental Vulnerability Model. The patient with dementia is more vulnerable to the environment and has a lower threshold where stimuli affect behavior. A stimulus that might be handled well by someone who is not suffering from Alzheimer's disease may be something a patient with dementia overreacts to because they are cognitively impaired.

Tools to Evaluate Behavior Problems in Dementia

While you probably wouldn't do this at home, your doctor or a nursing home facility might use one of these tools to see how much behavior is factoring into the care of the Alzheimer's patient. The most commonly used scale is called the Cohen Mansfield Agitation Inventory. This is a 29 item scale that looks at verbally agitated, physically nonaggressive and physically aggressive behavior. Each point is given from never exhibiting the behavior to exhibiting it several times an hour.

The Brief Agitation Scale is like the one above but it is shorter. There are about 10 items that ask many of the same questions as the Cohen Mansfield Agitation Inventory. The Pittsburgh Agitation Scale measures the severity of the agitation and does not measure frequency of episodes. It looks at motor agitation, aggressiveness and aberrant vocalizations.

The BEHAVE-AD scale is a four point scale that looks at the amount of paranoid delusions, delusional ideations, activity disturbances, aggressiveness, hallucinations, anxiety, affective disturbances and diurnal rhythm disturbances. It also rates the degree of phobias and provides a global rating of dangerousness and distress.

Many psychiatrists and neurologists use the Neuropsychiatric Inventory that looks at the severity, frequency and distress that occurs around behavioral disturbances. It looks at the emotional effects of the behavioral disruptions. There is a nursing home version of this inventory. Other helpful scales are the Overt Aggression Scale, the Behavior Rating Scale for Dementia, and the one used by caretakers, which is the Caretaker Obstreperous-Behavior Rating Assessment.

Taking a Close Look at Behaviors

There can be several reasons why the behavior of a person with Alzheimer's disease has deteriorated. Things that cause delirium, such as bladder infections, dehydration, hypoglycemia, hypoxia, electrolyte imbalance and drug toxicity can cause behavioral problems. For this reason, a urinalysis should be done along with electrolytes, drug levels, oxygen saturation and glucose levels should be assessed. Medications that mostly affect behavior are sedatives, steroids, narcotics and anticholinergics. Anticholinergics can make dementia worse so they should be looked at carefully. A medication review should be undertaken any time there is a behavioral change.

Depression, psychosis and anxiety need to be ruled out. It is estimated that delusions can be seen in 10-73 percent of those with dementia. Many delusions are related to suspiciousness, delusions of theft and personal threats of bodily harm. Delusions of misidentification are also possible and are seen 25 percent of the time. There can be hallucinations in up to 49 percent of cases of dementia. Among hallucinations, more are likely to be visual than auditory.

Sundowning is not believed to be from delirium but from darkness. It is due to aberrations in the individual's circadian rhythms and not to sensory inputs. Other behavioral outbursts can be related to the caregiver's behavior. If the caregiver is impatient or if the environment is frequently changed, there can be acting out of the behavior and this really isn't the fault of the person with dementia.

When dealing with outbursts of behavior, you need to ask yourself what exactly is the behavior that is being expressed. What were the circumstances of the behavioral event? What was the environment like? How frequent is the behavior and how long did the behavioral issue last? How bad was the behavior and what preceded it? Was the behavior issue associated with everyday activities of daily living? Does the patient seem to have control over the behaviors? Is the behavior related to a certain person or to too many people being present? What interaction precipitated the behavior and were there any events that predicted the oncoming presence of the behavior? Did the behavior serve any real purpose?

When you've asked these questions and answered them, you might find a way to reduce the incidence of behavioral issues. When you're not sure about what's going on, make an appointment with a geriatric psychiatrist who can make sure there isn't any underlying psychiatric problem going on and who can prescribe medications which might control behaviors. There may have been a preexisting psychiatric disorder that went untreated and that is now manifesting itself on top of dementia. The psychiatrist may ask if the patient was always nervous or if they had a history of violent behavior in the past. Past alcohol use may play a role in behaviors.

Treating Dementia-Related Behaviors

Treating dementia requires an approach that is both pharmacological and non-pharmacological. If the doctor decides to use medications, they should match the symptoms and should not just be given to sedate the Alzheimer's patient. In the same way, if the loved one is suffering from acute delirium, the doctor should find out if an infection such as a bladder infection is causing the problem. This problem should be treated with antibiotics instead of medications for psychosis.

In the same way, depression should be treated in dementia with antidepressants. Selective serotonin reuptake inhibitors or SSRIs are usually the first medications tried, especially Celexa because it doesn't have many reactions with other drugs. Older drugs for depression, like tricyclic antidepressants (amitriptyline and nortriptyline) should be avoided because they have a lot of side effects. The same is true of paroxetine. Wellbutrin can make seizures happen more often so you need to be careful to watch for seizures and stop the medication if necessary. Your doctor may use selegiline transdermal patches. This medication is called a monoamine oxidase inhibitor and works well when the patient refuses to take oral medicines. Long acting fluoxetine can be used on a once a week basis.

There are Alzheimer's drugs, like the acetylcholinesterase inhibitors, and memantine, that seem to act on depression in Alzheimer's patients, which is an effect much different from their ability to reduce dementia symptoms. Mirtaptine is a drug for depression that also improves appetite and sleep habits in those people who are both depressed and have dementia. In severe cases where no medication seems to help, electroconvulsive therapy can help and can reverse depressive symptoms.

Treating hallucinations and delusions is controversial. There is FDA warning that indicates a possible link with strokes and early mortality in patients who take these medications and have dementia. In addition, some studies indicate that antipsychotic medication in psychosis that comes out of dementia doesn't really work that well. They can cause weight gain, drug-induced Parkinson's disease and metabolic syndrome. Elderly people can get tardive dyskinesia from taking antipsychotic drugs as well.

Even so, antipsychotic drugs are helpful in some people. You just need to balance the risks and the benefits from taking these drugs and taper the drugs off once the behavior is in control. Before deciding to use antipsychotic medication in patients with dementia, ask yourself the following questions:

- Is the dementia patient bothered by these symptoms?

- Is the person being treated the caregiver or the dementia patient?

- Is the behavior disruptive to others?

- Will the behavior result in the patient having to move out of their home?

- Are there non-drug treatments that have yet to be tried?

If the patient also has bipolar disorder, they may need antipsychotics but the same precautions apply to them as they do to dementia patients that don't have bipolar disorder. They can use lithium, which is believed to protect one from dementia, carbamazepine, oxycarbazepine, and other drugs commonly used for bipolar disorder. Remember that lithium can be toxic to kidneys, especially in the elderly so the level must be measured periodically.

If a person with dementia is anxious, the usual anxiolytic medications like benzodiazepines are not used as a first line medication. This is because benzodiazepines can cause confusion and are a fall risk. Shorter acting medications are best, such as Ativan or lorazepam. The best choices are acetylcholinesterase inhibitors, memantine and SSRIs. Trazodone is not addictive and also works well to lessen anxiety. Quetiapine is also a good medication. Small amounts are given during the daytime hours and larger doses are given at night. Cautions similar to using antipsychotics need to be followed.

Sleep problem is a common problem among the elderly with behavior issues. Light therapy can be used to decrease the sundowning effect. The sleeping pills to keep in mind are those that don't cause grogginess and a fall risk in the morning. Ramelteon is a good sleeping medication that is a selective melatonin receptor agonist. It is safe and has no psychomotor effects on the elderly. It also does not affect their cognitive function. Two other medications that aren't indicated for sleep problems in the elderly but are used regularly include Trazodone and mirtazapine.

Helping Behavioral Issues without Using Drugs

There are things you can do to control behaviors that do not include medications. These things can be more important than just giving medications. Most interventions can be based on three models that lead to these behaviors in the first place. They include behaviors that relate to unmet needs; behaviors that need caregiver interventions and behaviors that need environmental interventions to reduce the behaviors.

Here are some behavioral interventions that can help:

- Replace eyeglasses, ill-fitting dentures and hearing aids to correct sensory deficits.
- Keep the physical environment comfortable, calm, and homelike. Surround the person with familiar possessions.
- Give the person regular daily structure with activities they enjoy, Try adult day care programs to enhance the activity level.
- Make sure regular wake and sleep patterns are met.
- Have safety measures installed to keep accidents away.
- Make sure there is respite for the caregiver.
- Have caregivers get educated on dementia and how to care for the dementia patient.
- Avoid confrontational behavior.
- Have caregivers skilled in taking care of daily living activities.
- Use adaptive clothing and devices to make sure bathing and dressing is simple.
- Have an experienced doctor.
- Get in touch with the local Alzheimer's Association.

Summary

Behavioral issues can be one of the top things that result in an Alzheimer's patient needing to see a doctor, go to a nursing home or be hospitalized. The causes of the behavior are often multifactorial; this makes the management of the problem multifaceted and challenging. The first thing a caregiver should do is use non-pharmacological interventions before turning to drug therapy.

Ideally, there should be a team of people that can help control the behaviors as they can often be organic, environmental, psychological and behavioral. When the behaviors are controlled, it often takes a great deal of stress off the caregiver. Think about causes of behaviors like bladder infections, low oxygen levels and other infections that can be treated and can reduce the behaviors that are simply secondary to a medical problem.

Chapter 7: The Nursing Home Environment

Many Alzheimer's disease patients live in nursing homes. In fact, there are about 232,000 Alzheimer's disease residents in the US today which account for 15.5 percent of all nursing home residents.

Making the decision to put your loved one in a nursing home is extremely difficult. On the other hand, caring for the same person in your home or their home can result in significant financial, personal and social sacrifices. Not every family has the funds or the resources to put in the effort to care for someone that is getting worse and worse over time.

When making your decision as to where your Alzheimer's loved one lives, think about the following issues:

- People with Alzheimer's disease need a structured environment that is both safe and healthy. If you cannot provide this at home, it may be better to transfer the individual to the nursing home.

- As the time goes on, the person may need increasing care. Decide when you have reached the ability to care for your loved one and, when that limit is reached, think about nursing home care.

- Can you find an adult day care facility or get part time help which can lengthen the time the individual is in the home.

- Know what your own personal physical and emotional health limits are. Don't sacrifice your own health for that of another person. You won't do anyone any good if you are too stressed out, depressed or physically ill.

- Remember that putting your relative in a nursing home doesn't represent failure on your part. It sometimes is a necessary part of life and it can be the best thing for the loved one.

Increasing Medical Needs

It's a fact of life that Alzheimer's disease will get worse over time and it will be harder and harder to care for them. Basic activities like toileting, dressing, bathing and eating need increasing amounts of help by the caregiver. The Alzheimer's patient has a more difficult time just getting around independently becomes impossible for them to do. Depending on the strength and stamina of the caregiver it might take more than one person to transfer the Alzheimer's patient from the bed to a wheelchair or vice versa.

Disruptive and dangerous behavior can develop and can be one of the biggest challenges of a caregiver. The loved one can break things or hit people. The dementia patient can emotionally berate the caregiver and it can become dangerous to be alone with them. It can become emotionally and physically impossible to care for the Alzheimer's patient.

Some people believe that they should continue to take care of their Alzheimer's spouse as long as the love one really recognizes who they are and knows where they are. The truth is that you can make use of the nursing home even when the Alzheimer's patient knows who they are. Going to the nursing home is a multi-variable thing to do and it depends on many factors.

Types of Long Term Care Facilities

There are several different long term care facilities you can choose from. They vary in their ability to care for the person with Alzheimer's disease. Many times, people refer to all long term care facilities as "nursing homes" when only some can be classified as "nursing homes". Here are some choices:

- **Assisted Living Facilities**. These are private homes that are set up like apartments. People live relatively independently but can get meals, bathing, grooming and dressing services on an as-needed basis. These are perfect places for those who have early Alzheimer's disease who is unable to live alone but who is able to function fairly well independently.

- **Residential Care Facilities**. These include retirement homes, board and care facilities, and foster care homes that provide more supervision that assisted living facilities. Residents get meals taken care of along with laundry, cleaning services and services around personal needs—all in a community setting. Medical care is not provided. This is a facility that is more appropriate for mild to moderate Alzheimer's disease. They tend to be cheaper than nursing homes but don't provide the daily nursing care some people with Alzheimer's disease need.

- **Nursing Homes**. These can provide complete nursing care 24 hours per day. The patient is provided with basically all aspects of personal care including medications, medical attention, meals, housing, laundry and personal cares. Social services are also provided. This is the most expensive kind of long term care and is usually where people go when they have advanced dementia, including Alzheimer's dementia.

- **Special Care Units or SCUs**. These are usually units within nursing homes that are specifically designed to manage patients with dementia. The staff has a special skill in caring for Alzheimer's patients and the environment tends to reflect the peacefulness and lack of chaos that the dementia patient needs.

- **Continuing Care Communities**. These are facilities that offer the widest range of care for the elderly. Everything from assisted living services to full nursing facility services are given and the dementia patient goes from area to area depending on the stage of their Alzheimer's disease.

- **Part time Care Options**. Some Alzheimer's dementia patients can get by at home but need part time paid care. This helps them stay in their home as long as is possible. The part time care can be adult daycare or it can be given at home. You can make use of a home health aide that takes care of personal cares and things like cleaning and bathing. You can also use a nurse that can help you with behavioral issues. The care can be done in your presence or can be done with the idea that they are providing respite care for you. It allows the caregiver some peace and the ability to get other jobs done.

- **Full Time Home Care**. While this can be an expensive option, you can hire people to take round the clock shifts to care for your loved one. It also involves you having to hire and manage a group of people on a 24 hour basis.

Making the Important Decision

The decision to give up home care of the Alzheimer's patient and instead think about something like nursing home placement is a difficult one. Often several family members must get together to discuss the issue and render a decision. The caregiver ultimately has the biggest voice and must take into account the medical facts and their own personal feelings. Ask yourself the following questions:

- Is the person's behavior disruptive or dangerous to those in your household?

- Is your own health at risk?

- Is the burden of giving care becoming greater?

- Do you have no one to help you?

- Is the person safe in your home?

- Is the environment controlled enough for the Alzheimer's patient?

- Does the resident/loved one have other medical issues that preclude staying at home?

- Might the individual decline too rapidly in the nursing home?

- Will the individual get enough attention in the nursing home?

- Will the individual get adequate care in the nursing home?

- Will you feel too much anxiety or guilt if you place the person in the nursing home?

- Does the facility have a long waiting list?

- Can the family afford nursing home care?

- Can you devote enough time to care-giving?

- Is there a long term care facility close to you?

After asking yourselves these questions, see if you can say on a scale of one to ten if you are leaning toward putting your relative in a nursing home (1) or if you are leaning toward keeping your relative at home (10). See a financial counselor or social worker at the nursing home to plan the ways in which you can pay for nursing home care. In some cases, the family can't pay for care and the person will go on General Assistance and Medicare to pay for the care they will receive in the nursing home.

A Look at Long Term Care

Long term care as it applies to people with Alzheimer's disease is a place where there are many medical, social and personal services that are designed to meet the emotional, physical and social needs of disabled people, those with long term illnesses and those with cognitive impairments. A place like a nursing home is often the best place for the affected individual to receive 24 hour care and helpful supervision.

There are two kinds of care you can expect to receive at one of these facilities for those who have Alzheimer's dementia. You can expect **basic care**. This is the care received that attends to the activities of daily living like grooming, bathing, medicines, dressing and supervision for safety reasons.

You can also expect **skilled care**. This needs one or more skilled registered nurses who can perform procedures and keep track of medication. It also includes the services that are given by trained health professionals, including physical therapy, occupational therapy, and respiratory therapy.

Typical services do vary from place to place but often include the patients' room and board, personal cares like toileting, bathing and dressing, monitoring of medication, emergency care provided on a 24 hour basis, and recreational and social activities.

Finding the Right Nursing Home

It can take time to find a nursing home that is suitable for a loved one with Alzheimer's disease. The search for a facility should take place a long time before you actually need the services. There can be waiting lists you might have to be on and finding out beforehand where you are going can easily take a lot of the worry and anxiety out of the actual move. Remember that the move will be stressful for everyone in the family.

As a family, you will want to think about what services you'd like to see. For example, do you want a facility that has a special care unit? Think about what kinds of help you'd like to see your loved one receive and how often you'd like them to receive it. Take a tour of every nursing home on your list to get an idea of the ambiance. Make sure to talk to one of the RNs about what it is like to work there. Talk to the social services person about what are the ways you will be able to fund the stay.

You should think about funding options long before you really need them. Know that Medicaid, Medicare, private insurance, long term care insurance and personal funds can be used to pay for the stay. Ask the social worker what kinds of monies they take and how long such funds are good for. For example, Medicare will only pay for a certain period of time and for certain services. Medicare is available for everyone over the age of 65; it I intended to cover for hospital stays regardless of the person's income but will pay for nursing services at a facility that has a Medicare license and has skilled care to offer the residents.

Medicaid comes from state and federal sources and is a health insurance program for low income Americans. Eligibility and covered services differ from state to state and not everyone is covered under this plan. Private insurance for long term care is something that you have to think about in advance of actually needing it. Every policy is unique in its eligibility requirements, benefits, costs, and restrictions.

Nursing Home Checklist

Take a look at this checklist. You should bring it along with you when you visit each nursing home. Some of the items will be more important to you than others but you must keep each thing in mind when searching for the perfect nursing home for a loved one that has Alzheimer's disease:

1. Do you get the level of care you are expecting, like skilled care or intermediate care?

2. Is the nursing facility properly licensed for what it does?

3. Is the nursing home administrator's license up to date?

4. Does the facility meet the state's fire regulations for things like fireproof doors, an evacuation plan, or a sprinkler system?

5. Are there specific visiting hours for the facility?

6. Does the facility have a policy regarding insurance and personal property?

7. Can the facility respond quickly to a medical emergency?

8. Does the facility have a current Medicare license?

9. What is the waiting period for admission to the nursing home?

10. Are there specific admission requirements that have to be met?

11. Are the fees competitive with other nearby facilities?

12. Have the fees gone up significantly in recent years?

13. Can you easily understand the fee structure?

14. What are their policies around billing, credit and payment?

15. Do different levels of services cost differing amounts of money?

16. Are the procedures for accounting and billing easy to understand?

17. Does the nursing home say what's covered in the basic fees?

18. What services are considered extra?

19. Does the nursing home take Medicaid, Medicare, Medicare Supplement Insurance, Supplemental Security Income, and other plans?

20. What is the policy around refunds and under what circumstances may a contract be terminated?

21. Does the staff write up a written plan of care for each resident?

22. What is the specific procedure for assessing a resident's needs?

23. How often are needs reassessed by the staff?

24. Does the staff receive education and experience in taking care of elderly patients?

25. Can the staff members easily meet a resident's scheduled and unscheduled needs?

26. Does it seem like the staff enjoys working and caring for the residents?

27. Are residents treated like individuals by the staff?

28. Can the staff members deal well with residents who suffer from problems with orientation, memory or judgment?

29. Is there a doctor that visits regularly to provide health checkups for the residents?

30. Do the residents seem comfortable and happy?

31. Do others, like relatives of other residents, speak well of the nursing home?

32. Is there a place where residents' rights are clearly posted?

33. Do you care for the appearance of the building and its grounds?

34. Is the décor home like and attractive?

35. Is it easy to follow the floor plan?

36. Do the hallways and doorway make room for walkers and wheelchairs?

37. Are there elevators on the floors?

38. Are there handrails along the hallway?

39. Do they have easy-to-reach shelves and drawers?

40. Are the carpets secured?

41. Are the floors mad out of non-skid material?

42. Is he indoor lighting natural and sufficient?

43. Is the residence free of odors and clean?

44. Is the nursing home properly cooled and heated?

45. What is the policy around where medications are stored and who gives them out?

46. How are visits with the occupational, physical, and speech therapists coordinated?

47. Is there a 24 hour availability of help for dressing, movement, bathing, toileting, eating, hygiene, grooming, and using the telephone?

48. Are there rooms for double and single occupancy?

49. Is there a 24 hour response system for each room/bed?

50. Are the bathrooms private?

51. Do the bathrooms fit walkers and wheelchairs?

52. Can residents bring in their own décor, including furniture?

53. Do all rooms have their own telephone? How are long distance phone calls handled?

54. Is there a special program for activities?

55. Are the activities posted for the residents?

56. Are these activities being participated in by the residents?

57. Is the food nutritionally balanced for each day of the week?

58. Is the food warm and tasty?

59. Can the residents have snacks?

60. Is drinking water always available?

61. Do residents eat in a common area or in their rooms?

62. Are there set mealtimes or do people eat when they want?

63. How do they handle special diets?

64. Are there staff members to help residents who can't feed themselves?

Summary

The decision to make use of a long term care facility such as a nursing home is a difficult one for the families of those who have a loved one with Alzheimer's disease. Usually the caregiver has exceeded their ability to care for their loved one and other arrangements need to be made. Hopefully, plans for such a time have been made in advance so that things like where to take the person to and how to pay for the services are worked out in advance.

Not all care facilities are alike. Some simply offer room and board with community support while others offer full services like 24 hour care, the services of an RN, and the services of occupational, physical and speech therapists. Some take Medicare and Medicaid, while others take only cash and private insurance money.

Nursing homes vary a lot with policies and levels of care. It pays to take the questions given above to each nursing home you are looking at so you can honestly compare their services and make decisions as to what things are more important to you than others.

Chapter 8: Caring for the Caregiver

Most caregivers are wonderful, selfless and amazing people who would do just about anything they can for the Alzheimer's person they are caring for. Unfortunately, providing this level of care, even for a loved one, takes a toll on the caregiver over time. Caregivers need to be alert to their level of stress and depression and must learn to find ways to take care of themselves, too. This sounds easy but, in fact, it is very difficult. They need support from others and they need to let go of the idea that they are the only one who can care for the loved one.

A caregiver can help their loved one with daily needs such as going to physician's appointments, picking up medicines and making meals. The often help the person with dementia cope with their emotional needs. There are interchanges where the loved one needs to

vent to the caregiver his or her anger or sadness. The caregiver can help with their loved
one's confusion.

When the caregiver provides care, it is
normal to put his/her own feelings and needs
aside. If this has to happen for a long period of
time, it is not good for the health of the caregiver. As a care giver, you need to take care of
your needs, too. If you fail to do this, you can
be unable to care for others.

These are the feelings you might be dealing with:

- **Guilt**. Feels of guilt are common. You
  might feel as though you aren't providing enough help or feel guilty because
  you are healthy and your loved ones
  are not.

- **Grief**. You may be having strong feelings of loss over your loved ones lack of
  health or it might be the loss of the day
  to day life you once shared with your
  loved one who now has Alzheimer's
  disease.

- **Loneliness**. It is possible to feel lonely,
  even if there are many people around
  you. You might have your loved one

around you but be unable to have meaningful conversation with them.

- **Fear**. You may not know what the future holds and might be scared of what will happen to you and your loved one.

- **Sadness**. Sadness is normal. If sadness lasts for more than two weeks and if it keeps you from doing normal activities, you may have depression and may need to see a doctor.

- **Anger**. You can be angry at yourself, your loved one, or with other family members. Anger can be directed at the fact that your loved one has Alzheimer's disease. This feeling can come out of feeling panicked, fearful or distressed.

So what kinds of things may help you? You can talk to a family member, priest, friend pastor or therapist about your feelings. You might also need to talk to your doctor, who understands your position and what you are going through.

Think about these things as you provide care to a loved one with Alzheimer's disease:

- Remember that no one is perfect and everyone makes mistakes, especially when they have a lot on their minds.

- Don't be afraid to cry or to express how you really feel. You do not have to be "cheerful" when you don't really feel that way. It is perfectly okay to show that you are upset or sad.

- Let the little things go. Don't do chores if you are tired and take your time doing things that are really worth the energy and time.

- Be reminded that you are doing the best you can given your circumstances.

- Spend some time by yourself to really think about your feelings. It is common to feel overwhelmed and stress out, worried about your loved one.

- Try to share how you feel with any other person who can help you.

- Know that everyone is different and their reactions will differ. All of your feelings are completely valid and worth expressing. There is no right way to feel in these circumstances.

Many emotions come to the surface because of all the stressors the caregiver must deal with. The feelings that come up can be directed inward or can be directed at the person who is ill. It can also be directed at other family members who may or may not be pulling their weight. As these emotions can be pent up and can make the caregiver sick, it is important to let the emotions out through expressing oneself. Whether you are near tears or ready to lash out in anger, find an outlet for these difficult emotions. Take the time, too, to list the things in life that you are grateful for.

Be sure to find sources to talk to. It can be an individual therapist or psychologist; it can also be a support group for caregivers of Alzheimer's patients. Talking to someone who shares your burden is a good idea when you are dealing with long term care of a loved one. If you think you are depressed, talk to your family doctor or a psychiatrist about getting on an antidepressant.

Know your limitations, what triggers you and what your expectations are around your situation. Take the time to figure out when your most negative emotions show up. Do you have reasonable expectations of being a caregiver? Which situations try your patients the most? Remember that it is the disease acting up and not your loved one. They cannot help it. Worrying over those things over which you have no control doesn't really help things. Focus on the little things that go on in your life that give you pleasure. Caregiving without pleasure at least some of the time will certainly lead to ill feelings and possibly anxiety and depression.

Things you can do:

It pays to think ahead and do things that will make your life easier as you care for a loved one with Alzheimer's disease. These are some things you can do:

- **Make a Schedule**. Schedules take a little bit of time to do but make things much easier when it comes to caring for an Alzheimer's patient. Keep track of doctors' appointments, visitor times and times for doing activities of daily living. You might find blocks of time with nothing in it so that you can use that time for yourself to get your hair cut or just relax for a little bit. See if you can find blocks of time in which another relative or friend can come in and give you some respite care.

- **Make time for personal time away from your home**. You really must get away sometime, especially if the one you care for lives with you. You can find time to go out to dinner with friends or take your grandkids or children with you to a movie. This time away is truly a fresh breath of air that you need in order to revive the strength you need to do the work you do. Consider hiring someone on a temporary basis to provide you respite care.

- **Find personal time in your home**. Find a quiet place in your house to read or watch television by yourself. You can even participate in prayer, playing a musical instrument, meditation or writing/journaling. The more you can do to relax and refresh yourself, the better the caregiver you will be. Remember that this is your home and it should feel comforting to you as well.

- **Find time for exercise**. Exercise is one of the more important things you can do to handle the stress you're under. Even if you can exercise 15 minutes per day at least three times per week can be enough exercise to relieve stress. If you can't get outside, buy a treadmill that you can sneak in an exercise program with. In addition, getting regular exercise has been found to delay the onset of Alzheimer's disease and other types of dementia.

- **Think about meaningful time together**. Just because there are cognitive differences between you and your loved one doesn't mean that you can't spend quality time together. Select an activity like baking, singing to the radio, watching TV or going out to a park that you both can enjoy and share together. These kinds of moments keep you from burning out from caregiving.

When you have a loved one that has been diagnosed with Alzheimer's disease, understand that your friends or other family members may not realize what is happening in your home. This may lead to frustration and the need to constantly have to explain what's going on to other members of the family. Take the time to educate your loved ones about the course of dementia so they understand that things will change over time and the relative they know now might not be the same when they next see them.

Keep specific times or tasks that other family members can do and approach them with the ideas you have come up with. See if they can take the ill family member to doctors' appointments or watch the family member so you can get groceries or just to have a break. If there are family members that live far away, you could ask them to stay for a couple of days so they can give you a break and so you have people to talk to besides your loved one with dementia. You might be surprised at who will help you out when it comes to caring for your loved one. In many cases, it is their loved one, too.

Dealing with Special Events and Holidays

Holidays can be especially awkward for individuals who have dementia. Family members and other visitors come and go and there are unfamiliar sights and sounds—lots of activity and children—all things that can increase the confusion and add to the possibility of emotional outbursts in the elderly person with dementia. Visitors may express dismay at the changes they observe in the dementia patient. Traditions may have to be changed. In fact, there are things that you can do that can make holidays and family gatherings go as smoothly as possible.

- Try to make the gatherings as small and intimate as possible.

- Prepare your visitors in advance so they know what to expect from the loved one.

- Keep on doing familiar traditions and do them in familiar settings.

- Let the person with dementia participate to the degree they can.

Depression is a common phenomenon among elderly people and this can get worse around the time of the holidays. The dementia patient may feel lost and disoriented during the holidays; they may feel feelings of sadness.

It's possible they miss holidays of long ago that cannot be the same anymore. They might not recognize all the family members and may feel like someone should be there that's not there anymore. Caregivers may feel similar losses because they know that holidays are not the same and won't ever be the same again. Dealing with hard emotions can challenge the ideal of a perfect holiday. It helps to speak with your doctor before the holidays occur, especially if you suspect either one of you will struggle with depression.

It's common for those with dementia to feel less than enthusiastic around the holidays. This might be completely different from the caregivers who feel nostalgic around past holidays. Try to keep traditions going to the best of your ability so that all family members get to participate to the best of their ability. Some traditions might have to be modified or stopped altogether if they become too dangerous to continue. The holiday traditions can disrupt the usual routines for the elderly person so be prepared to smooth things over.

You can travel with a person with dementia but it is tricky to do and may not be possible if the individual has a lot of outbursts.

Special Tips for a Happy Holiday

One thing you can do is to revise your traditions so that everyone can participate. Think of simple, repetitive tasks that are safe for everyone to do and that can be done with the loved one with Alzheimer's disease. Try these holiday activities:

- String garland with natural items
- Make wreaths
- Make paper chains
- Make special photo albums
- Bake cookies together
- Write greeting cards out for loved ones
- Read holiday stories or stories from the Bible

Keep your holiday expectations in line with what is realistic. You may not have the perfect family gathering but you can still get together and enjoy the holiday time in different ways. You can even enjoy a walk together, if weather permits. Keep to your regular schedules as best you can and make sure the most chaotic family times together are during times when the Alzheimer's patient is the calmest. Be sure to take care of yourself during this challenging yet exciting time.

Support Groups

Joining a support group for caregivers of those with Alzheimer's disease is a smart choice and a way to get information and inspiration from others who are in a similar situation. There are support groups put on by your local Alzheimer's Association or by the Area Agency on Aging programs. These groups tend to be held around once per month for about 1 to 2 hours and are located at nearby hospitals, churches or senior centers.

Groups tend to be run by a skilled moderator and give everyone the chance to introduce themselves and to talk about their situation. Caregivers can then discuss problems they all have in common and can problem-solve their difficulties. They often share similar stories and comfort one another when thing aren't going well. They might invite some guest speakers that can talk about aspects of Alzheimer's disease. As a caregiver, you can participate as much or as little as you feel comfortable. Most, on the other hand, enjoy sharing their tory and getting advice from people who understand completely what you are going through. The support and encouragement you get from others in the support group can make all the difference between feeling positive about your role as caregiver and feeling depressed.

Summary

You care best for your loved one with Alzheimer's disease when you learn to take time for yourself. Whether it be getting respite care, joining an Alzheimer's support group or just taking time for yourself, these are things that can make the whole experience bearable. If you live with your Alzheimer's person, you are subjected to their 24 hour needs and issues. This can bear on anyone so that anxiety and depression become common among caregivers.

As a caregiver, you need to know your limitations and not go too far past their boundaries. Think about things like exercise, meditation, prayer and reading as ways to improve your stamina and feel more relaxed.

Holidays can be especially stressful as your regular routine is broken up. Take the time to keep those holiday traditions that can be kept and let go of those that no longer fit with your lifestyle.

Conclusion

Caregivers are selfless, amazing people who have a big job to do when it means taking care of an Alzheimer's loved one. They often are responsible for making meals, dressing, taking care of doctors' appointments, giving medications, bathing, grooming and feeding the person with dementia.

Alzheimer's disease has no known cause. Researchers have found amyloid plaques and neurofibrillary tangles in the brains of Alzheimer's patients and these findings can be seen even before symptoms develop using special technology that highlights the brain. It can take a decade or more to actually develop symptoms.

There are several stages to Alzheimer's disease. They usually begin with mild memory loss that can be written off to old age and progress to where the patient is nonverbal and cannot recognize any family members.

Motor skills decline so the patient becomes wheelchair bound or bed bound. These stages altogether take about ten years.

There is an early onset type of Alzheimer's disease that begins between 30 to 60 years of age. It appears to be hereditary. Late onset dementia usually begins after age 60 and increases in frequency so that a large proportion of patients have the disease by age 85.

You as caregiver must be in tune with the needs and wishes of the loved one you care for, while caring for yourself. A caregiver can be a spouse, a child or grandchild of the person with Alzheimer's disease. They often have problems with work and financial difficulties because of the time they must spend with the Alzheimer's patient.

Safety is very important when taking care of someone with dementia. There are "baby proofing" things you must do to keep the person you are caring for safe. In some cases, it comes to putting external locks on the inside of the home so that the person cannot escape. There are issues around driving that need to be addressed before they come up.

The unpaid caregiver is usually a relative of the Alzheimer's patient. They often devote many hours a week to caring for the person with dementia. Caregivers need to learn how to care for themselves by taking part in an Alzheimer's support group, talking to a psychologist or talking to a pastor about the feelings and issues that are going on.

The caregiver must be able to deal with eating issues in the elderly. They often have a decreased internal thirst so they have problems swallowing dry food. There are tricks the caregiver can utilize to help the Alzheimer's patient swallow and eat better.

Behavioral problems, including delusions and hallucinations are common in Alzheimer's disease. It is up to the caregiver and the doctor to decide whether to medicate the behaviors or whether to handle them with behavioral modification.

If the cares become too difficult, the caregiver and the family need to think about a long term care facility, such as a nursing home. This requires asking a lot of questions about the nursing homes being looked at so that the nursing home of choice meets the patient's needs.

Finally, the caregiver needs looking after, too. This means family members must gather together to pitch in and provide respite care for the caregiver. If this doesn't happen, the

caregiver can become ill and can become depressed.